Back to Basics

A Fitness Instructors Guide to Healthy Living

Author:

Jeri Shivers,

AFAA, FiTOUR - Certified Group Exercise & Mat Pilates Instructor

Contents

Part One: Strategies for Success - What works

    A. Commitment
    B. Set Goals
    C. Get Support but Take Responsibility
    D. Calorie Intake, What are you eating
    E. Exercise
    F. Healthy Lifestyle

Part Two: Food Pyramid aka MyPlate

    A. Understanding Servings

Part Three: Portion Size and Control

    A. Read the label
    B. What does it look like?

Part Four: What is Metabolism?

    A. How it works

Part Five: "Would you like to Super-Size that?"

    A. Strategies for eating out

Part Six: Conclusion

    A. Tips and Tricks

Bonus: Snack Choices under 150 Calories, Skinny Cocktails, Daily Exercises and food groups

I dedicate this book to the women
who have stayed with me through all the dry
spells and supported me all these years.

Thank you

Introduction

This year in September I turn 50. It marks a 10 year milestone as a Group Exercise instructor and 6 years as a Mat Pilates instructor. Both certifications of which I obtained to maintain my commitment to maintaining my weight as I got older.

The small rural town where I live had no instructors so the only competition I had was the lazy life styles people tend to live. It has been an exciting journey with my faithful followers. Followers that stayed with me through a hysterectomy that required 12 weeks of recovery. When I was ready to come back, so were they.

I'm not a physician, a nurse or a nutritionist. I am one women that had a desire to change her attitude, appearance and wellbeing. The information in the following pages are based on my sole research, study and personal experience. There are things in my 10 years as an instructor that I have seen work and there are things that I have seen that don't work. I have given advice and offered encouragement throughout the years; some which was taken and some which was not.

One thing stands unchanged; maintaining a healthy life is not rocket science! It's pretty basic; exercise, good nutrition and happiness. As we age, our exercise modality may change and our caloric needs may change, but the basic concept remains the same. There is no magic pill, drink or shake that is a miracle fix.

The strategies and suggestions in this book are guidelines I have used for years with success. They are basic guidelines adaptable by anyone.

As we age our body changes and the guidelines allow for setting new goals and making new commitments to maintain a healthy life at any age.

Part One:
Strategies for Success
What works

A. Make a commitment - A healthy lifestyle requires commitment and focus. No one can make you eat healthy or exercise; no one but YOU. First and foremost, it must be a change that pleases you.

Are you ready to make permanent changes?

B. Set attainable goals - Set goals that are realistic for you. It's easier to attain "process goals", such as "I will exercise 3 days a week" or "I will cut 200 calories a day by eliminating one soft drink." (or any other weakness). Take this slow so it can be maintained.

Take baby steps.

C. Get support - Only you can take responsibility of your own actions. But that doesn't mean you don't need encouragement from family and friends. If your family doesn't want to join you in your quest (but you should try to include them, they will benefit as well) to a healthier life, find a friend that has similar goals and give each other encouragement.

Stick together!

D. What are you eating? - Adopting new eating habits that include less calories promotes healthier living and weight loss. Don't confuse fewer calories with giving up on taste, satisfaction or the things you love. One way to lower calorie intake is to eat more fruits and veggies. Cutting back calories is easier if you focus on limiting fats; such as butter, margarine and oils. Don't limit yourself to certain foods, you will just set yourself up for failure. Eat the things you enjoy; this is where portion control plays its part.

Moderation, moderation, moderation!! Nothing should be off limits.

E. Move your body - Eating healthier alone can help with weight loss, but if you move your body aka "exercise" for 20 to 30 minutes on most days you can double your rate of weight loss. If your goal is to simply maintain a healthy weight, exercise is still an important part of a healthy lifestyle. It helps control diabetes, heart disease and osteoporosis. Little spurts of exercise throughout the day add up; take the stairs when possible, park far out into the parking lot and save the up close parking spaces for the people who need them. Choose a modality that inspires you to exercise. If you enjoy dancing, try a salsa class or a Zumba class. Walking and swimming are excellent lo-impact cardio activities and for stretching, toning and conditioning try a Pilates or Yoga session.

Move it, move it, move it!!

F. Lifestyle Changes - It's not enough to make these changes for only a few weeks or months. It has to be for a life time. Lifestyle changes start by taking an honest look at your eating habits and daily routine. Once you've identified your challenges, work out a strategy to obtain your goals of gradually changing your habits and your attitude. Admitting and recognizing your challenges is the first step to achieving your goals. It won't always be easy; you will have days of set-backs but don't beat yourself up. Start anew the next day. Believe me, it doesn't happen overnight, but if you will stick to your new changes and make them habits, the results will be worth it.

When I first began my journey to a healthier me, the first thing I did was buy a spiral notebook and wrote down what it was I wanted to accomplish – GOALS.

Then I wrote down what things could possibly hinder or get in the way of my plans. Such as; a luncheon meeting, a child's sporting event or concert, or going out of town. These things have the potential of sabotaging an eating plan or exercise class, but they can be modified. I made plans to try to work around or work with these events and plan a head. It really wasn't hard, but there are times you just can't make it happen and that's ok.

Set some goals. Make a plan. Write it down.

Part Two:
Food Pyramid
aka
MyPlate

Guidelines for choosing foods are widely represented in various food pyramids. The triangular shape of the pyramid shows you where to focus when selecting food. Foods to eat the most of create the base of the pyramid, and foods to eat in smaller amounts or more sparingly are shown farther up the pyramid.

June 1st, 2011, the standard food pyramid was replaced with a color coded plate (MyPlate.gov). Which makes sense, after all we eat off plates, right? The new plate represents what portions of the plate should be filled with what foods. If you go to the web-site it encourages you to fill half your plate with fruits and veggies, the other half with grains and protein. It advises limiting your sodium laden foods and avoid oversized portions. To get serving sizes you must go on the web-site and customize "your plate".

It looks easy enough, but I've gotten use to "serving numbers" and "serving sizes". I've lived by the pyramid for years. So you should evaluate and choose the method that best works for you.
Here are the most recent serving sizes based on USDA web-site:

Bread, cereal, rice and pasta group - 6 to 11 servings. A serving is 1 ounce.
Veggies group - 3 to 5 servings. A serving is ½ cup.
Fruit group - 2 to 4 servings. A serving is ½ cup.
Milk, yogurt and cheese group - 2 to 3 servings. A serving is ½ cup or 4 ounces
Meat, poultry, fish, eggs, beans and nuts group - 2 to 3 servings. A serving is 6 ounces
Fats, oils and sweets - sparingly, 2 to 6 teaspoons. A serving is 1 teaspoon.

Eating healthy takes a little preparation, but once in the habit it's just like getting up and getting dressed; it just becomes part of your daily routine.

Plan healthy meals and snacks using recommended food servings. Focus on foods at the base of the pyramid or larger portion of the "plate" - veggies, fruits and whole grains. Don't shy away from carbs, these are the fuels that give us energy, but do keep in mind moderation and portion control.

Choose a variety of foods from each food group. This ensures you get all the calories, protein, vitamins, fiber and nutrients you need.

Adapt the plan to the things you like, after all this is YOUR plan. It doesn't mean you can't have a flour tortilla, just exchange your regular flour tortilla for a low carb wheat tortilla. If you don't like apples, eat strawberries or blueberries.

They're loaded with fiber and antioxidants. Save yourself some time and buy them in your frozen food section already prepared. They are great frozen!!

Become familiar with the serving sizes of each food group. Read, read, read the labels!!
Spread out the food servings throughout your day. Try to include at least one serving from most food groups at each meal. Make the most of what you eat by choosing nutrient-rich foods with in each group. If you have an intolerance to certain foods, choose other foods that supply you the nutrients found in those foods. Chances are you already know what they are!!

Stay flexible and adjust your food serving goals as necessary. You know there will be times you can't eat according to your plan, do the best you can by choosing the healthiest things available. You can get back on track tomorrow.

For many years I kept track of things in a spiral notebook. I found it kept me true to myself. If I was getting close to reaching my daily calorie intake, then I would adjust my servings. It was all right there in black and white. In more recent years I found a great web-site that took all the hard work out of writing down calories, fat grams, fiber grams and carbs. You just entered the food item and serving size and it calculated it for you. Saved me a lot of time. Today there are a number of useful web-site tools out there, just Google it and you will see. But if you're new to food logs go check out *www.fatsecret.com.*

Along with logging everything I ate, I asked myself these things every day:

> *Did you eat out?*
> *Did you super-size?*
> *Did you drink more than 1 soda today?*
> *Did you eat any candy today?*
> *How many fruits servings did you eat today?*
> *How many veggie servings did you eat today?*
> *How many glasses of water did you drink today?*
> *Did you encounter any roadblocks?*
> *Did you exercise today?*

Start your log TODAY!!

Part Three:
Portion Size and Control
Read the labels

Maintaining, controlling or losing weight calls for more than just choosing a healthy variety of foods. It also calls for looking at how much and how often we eat. You need to look at using serving sizes to help you eat just enough.

What is the difference between a portion and a serving?

A "portion", as defined by *www.merriam-webster.com/dictionary*; an individual's part or share of something.

As we all know portions come in all shapes and sizes. What is a portion of pasta at home is different than a portion of pasta at an Italian restaurant.

A "serving" is the amount of food listed on the items Nutrition Facts label. Sometimes, the portion size and serving size match; but often times they do not. It is a quick way of letting you know what the calories and nutrients are in a certain amount of food.

The US Food and Drug Administration Nutrition Facts information is printed on most packaged foods. It tells you how many calories and how much fat, carbohydrates, sodium and other nutrients are available in one serving of food. Most packaged food contains more than a single serving. The serving sizes that appear on food labels are based on FDA-established lists of foods.

The "portion" size that you are used to eating may be equal to two or three standard servings. Take a look at the nutritional facts, you may eat two servings of canned green beans and that's ok, but look at the Mac and Cheese box, weigh the values; is two servings worth the doubling of calories and fat in it? I would think not!!

Read the labels, to see how many servings a package has. Check the "servings per container/package" listed on the Nutrition Facts, you may be surprised what you read. Small containers often have more than one serving in them. Take a pint of ice cream for example, most have 4 servings. Let's look at Ben & Jerry's Vanilla Heath Bar Crunch.

Servings per container - 4 - ½ cup servings
290 calories, per SERVING
19 grams of fat, per SERVING
28 grams of carbs, per SERVING
27 rams of sugar, per SERVING

Eat the whole pint and holy moly, you do the math!! Learn to recognize standard serving sizes.

If you are a more visual person, it may help you to compare food portions to everyday objects. Below are some suggestions that I have found are awfully close to the actual measurement. Learn them, the do come in handy.

1 cup = baseball
½ cup = light bulb
¼ cup = golf ball
2 tablespoons = ping pong ball
1 tablespoon = poker chip
6 ounces of meat or fish = a deck of cards
1 ounce of cheese = 3 dice
1 – 6 inch pancake = 1 CD
1/3 cup of rice or pasta = ½ a tennis ball
Medium size apple = a tennis ball
Slice of cornbread = a bar of soap

Don't panic, you don't have to measure and count for the rest of your life, but I do recommend you do it long enough to recognize a typical serving size. I still do it.

Part Four:
Metabolism
What's all the hype?

What is metabolism?

As defined by www.merriam-webster.com/dictionary ; the chemical changes in living cells by which energy is provided for vital processes and activities and new material is assimilated.

WHAT???

Metabolism has always been a buzzword in the fitness world, but following advice can be tricky. As we get older our metabolism slows down so we look for that one secret weapon that helps boost that calorie burn and keep those unwanted pounds at bay. Do we lift more weights? Do more cardio? Eat special food?

It has been cited that green tea is a metabolism booster, but the truth is, recent studies show that it has no bearing on increased metabolism or calorie burning effects. However it does have other health benefits, so if green tea is your thing, by all means keep drinking it. But don't count on it torching calories by boosting your metabolism.

Another common theory to boosting metabolism is eating 6 small meals a day as opposed to eating 3 large meals. There is no proven research to this. However, what this strategy does do is works as a weight control mechanism for many people; it helps keep blood sugar in check and keeps you from feeling hungry. So if this is your strategy, do it to keep from bingeing and not to boost metabolism.

Bottom line; exercise (the energy by which chemical changes occur) keeps the metabolism going. The trick is finding your zone of intensity that your body burns calories. That means any exercise regimen that incorporates cardio with strengthening and toning. If you enjoy exercising alone, walking or jogging may be your modality. If keeping you committed means exercising with a group, join an aerobics class or take dance lessons. Strengthening and toning are vitally important as well. Again choose you preferred modality; lift weights, join a Pilates or Yoga class or do a stretching DVD in your living room.

The fitter you become, the more calories you burn. Well-conditioned muscles burn more than three times the calories as opposed to a pound of fat. The catch is to use resistance or a weight heavy enough to challenge the muscle by the last rep. Wimpy weights need not apply!

So..............................read your labels, man your portions, log your food and exercise most days of the week. It's that simple.

Part Five:
Would you like to Super-Size that?
Strategies for eating out

Are you a fast food fiend?

Notorious for; just grabbing something on the way home, too tired to cook or plain just don't want to. Well, all that comes at a price.

A caloric price.

A typical burrito has about 700 calories and 26 grams of fat; a Chinese chicken dish, like Kung Pao, about 1000 calories and loaded with sodium.

Does that mean you can't eat out? Absolutely not! But you must be educated to the fast food menus. All the leading chains have nutritional pamphlets right in their joints. But if you can't find them there, look them up on the web.

Study them. Learn the nutritional values and make wise choices.

Stop being so "value-minded" and for heaven sakes don't "Super-Size" it just because it's .50 cents more! Ok, so you can get double the fries, but you get double the calories and the fat as well. No, no, no!!

Learn to make your own "fast food". Like fish tacos or chicken quesadillas. Their quick and easy and taste just as good with a lot less calories and fat.

Ok ladies, I know you enjoy a "girls night" out, but skip the fruity cocktails. A single frozen Margarita can have a whopping 365 calories; and who can stop at just one. Then there's the chips and salsa, oh my!! Instead take the party to someone's house and mix up a batch of "skinny" margaritas, cutting the calories almost by 75 percent. That's worth moving the party for. My girlfriends and I get together twice a month at a friend's house, she makes the best "skinny" margaritas. We don't sabotage our healthy eating habits and we have a great time!!

I'm not a fast food junkie, but if you must; here are some better choices (straight off their nutritional pamphlet).

> *McDonald McChicken - 370 cals, 16g fat*
> *Taco Bell Fresco Style Crunchy Taco - 150 cals, 7g fat*
> *Taco Bell Fresco Style Grilled Steak Soft Taco - 170 cals, 5g fat*
> *Pizza Hut 12" Diced Chicken, Red Onion and Green Pepper; 2 slices - 340 cals, 9g fat*
> *Pizza Hut 12" Veggie Lovers Hand Tossed Pizza; 1 slice - 220 cals, 6g fat*
> *Wendy's Jr. Hamburger - 280 cals, 9g fat*
> *Wendy's Large Chili - 330 cals, 9g fat*
> *Wendy's Ultimate Chicken Grill - 330 cals, 9g fat*

If something sweet is what you need, try these:

> *McDonald Vanilla Ice Cream Cone (it's reduced fat) - 150 cals, 3.5g fat*
> *Taco Bell Cinnamon Twists - 160 cals, 5g fat*
> *Wendy's Jr. Frosty - 160 cals, 4g fat*
> *KFC Lil' Bucket Strawberry Shortcake - 200 cals, 6g fat*
> *Pizza Hut Cherry Dessert Pizza: 1 slice - 240 cals, 3.5g fat*
> *KFC Lemon Meringue Pie Slice - 240 cals, 9g fat*

I know you can't eat at home every night and I know the best laid plans sometimes fail, but eating at home is the best option for a healthy meal plan.

Americans spend $117 billion a year on fast food (Womens Health Magazine June 2014). Money that could otherwise go a long way toward buying things that might actually improve our health. Break out that crock-pot that's got the dust all over it and then google "low-fat crock pot recipes" you'll be amazed at what you find. A little planning goes a long ways.

Part Six:
Conclusion
Tips and Tricks

As we age it becomes harder and harder to maintain our weight; but it can be done with a little time and commitment - eat right!

Build around a foundation of fruits, veggies, whole grains, low fat dairy and proteins. It's pretty basic.

Don't deny yourself the foods you love..remember moderation.

Don't fear fat; it helps you feel satisfied. So don't make everything "low fat".

Remember to maintain your caloric intake. The average women should not consume less than 1,200 calories a day. You may be cutting out vital nutrients your body needs. You have to eat to lose weight; 3 meals and 2 snacks a day or 6 small meals a day, whichever method works for you (6 small meals is my preference).

Eat your breakfast! Statistics show oatmeal can lower your risk of heart disease, one of the number one causes of death in women. Start your day off right.

If you find it hard to keep track of your daily intake try logging in a journal. If journaling is not your cup of tea, there are a number of inter-net web-sites that can help you log your food and exercise, keeping track of calories consumed and calories burned. There are also a number of meal plan programs to help you get all your food groups consumed.

I am not endorsing any products; but two of my favorites that I have been successful with are: www.fatsecret.com and the 21-day Beach Body Meal Plan. Don't let the name scare you away, the program utilizes color coded containers identifying the different food groups and a chart for keeping track of the number of servings consumed. The concept and plan is simple and easy to follow. Be true to yourself and log everything.

Educate yourself; read, read, read. Food labels are a wealth of information. Compare and make educated choices.

Stay hydrated and restrict your salt intake. Many times weight gain is due to fluid retention. Drink 8, 8 ounce glasses of water a day and flush out the excess salt and fluid.

Choose low-fat dairy products, it can reduce body fat by 70 percent.

Mix things up!! Don't eat the same things every day, add variety; make it interesting and enjoyable. Go out with the "girls" or your guy, don't deny yourself the things you love and bring you joy. Remember; it's all in moderation.

Move......................your......................body!!

Exercise is key. Do something most days of the week. Mix it up. Walk, jog, swim, take a Pilates class, take a dance class, yoga, stretching; the options are endless. Choosing something you enjoy will keep you going back.

I have found that not only does exercise help with maintaining a healthy weight, it also helps with depression and the many effects of menopause.

Never say, "Never"..

> *I'm never eating chocolate............*
> *I'm never eating ice cream......................*
> *I'm never eating bread.........................*

Hello???? Can you say, "binge"?? You should never make anything completely off limits. That one thing will be the very thing you will want every day. Remember moderation in the foods that you love.

Attitude is everything. Set attainable goals for yourself. Unreasonable expectations are discouraging and the main reason people give up on change. Don't say, "I'm losing 20 pounds in 2 weeks." That's ludicrous!! And highly unreasonable. Instead tell yourself, "I'm cutting my calorie intake by 300 calories a day and going to Pilates class 3 times a week." Anyone can do that! 300 calories a day could be one serving of Mac and Cheese!! Don't set yourself up for failure.

Be true to yourself.

Make healthy changes and reap the lifelong benefits.

Bonus:
Snack Choices under 150 Calories
Skinny Cocktails
Exercises for Any Body
Healthy Suggestions from each
Food Group

Snack Choices under 150 Calories

Skinny Cow Vanilla Ice Cream Sandwich
½ ounce of Raisins and 2 tablespoons of soy nuts
10 ounces of light yogurt smoothie
6 ounces Greek yogurt (Chobani makes a 100 calorie one with 12g protein and 5g fiber)
14 almonds and a small apple
½ cup Raspberry Sorbet
12 ounces Caramel Frappuccino Light (sans the whip cream)
1 ounce of chocolate covered almonds
18 soy chips
Fage 0% greek yogurt and ¼ cup blueberries
100 calorie mini bag popcorn
1 ounce string cheese and 4 wheat grain crackers
¼ cup Hummus and ½ cup baby carrots
Root beer float - ½ cup frozen vanilla yogurt and 12 ounces Diet Root Beer
Kellog's Nutri-Grain Fruit & Oat Harvest Bars Blueberry Bliss
Welch's PB&J Snacks - Creamy Concord Grape
Dannon Oikos Strawberry Greek Frozen Yogurt
Sargento Natural Extra Sharp Cheddar Cheese Sticks
Smartfood Delight Popcorn Sea Salt
Kashi All Natural Hummus Crisps Sundried Tomato Basil & Feta

The Skinny on Cocktails

I love a cool cocktail as much as the next girl, but let's face it they aren't on the list of "most nutritious for you". But there are options.

Always remember..............................moderation.

Be very wary with your alcoholic beverages. Alcoholic consumption can play a large part in weight gain. So if you find you're eating healthy and exercising, but still have that little "tummy pudge", check your cocktail consumption. It can change your weight drastically.

Per 8 ounce serving, typical restaurant style

White Wine Spritzer - 121 calories, 1.5g sugar
Mint Julep - 140 calories, 3g sugar
Rum Punch - 206 calories, 30g sugar
Cosmopolitan - 217 calories, 15g sugar
Frozen Margarita - 365 calories, 12 sugar

Try these "skinnies" :

Budwieser Select 55 - 55 calories
Michelob Catus Lime - 95 calories
Michelob Ultra - 90 calories
Jose Cuervo Light Margarita with Cuervo Gold - 95 calories, 0g sugar (4 oz serving)
Chi-Chi Skinny Margarita Mix - 95 calories, 0g sugar (4 oz serving)

Mix your own "skinnies":

Skinny 'Rita: about 74 calories (makes two 8 oz servings)

- 1 packet Limeade drink mix (like Crystal Light) mix according to packet (try Club Soda)
- 3 ounces of Tequila
- Lime wedges
- Salt for rimming the glass (optional, sparingly)

Mix first two ingredients, pour over ice, garnish and serve.

Strawberry Mint Sangria: about 100 calories

- ½ cup Red Wine (4 oz) (try Skinny Girl)
- ½ cup Club Soda (4 oz)
- 2 Strawberries
- 2-3 mint leaves
- 1 Splenda packet
- Add any fruit you have - grapes, oranges, limes

Chop mint leaves in small pieces, mash mint and strawberries together. Layer mint and strawberries in bottom of glass, add other ingredients, stir gently. Chill and serve

Peach Fizz

- 1 cup Club Soda or Diet Lemon Lime Soda
- 1.5 oz Peach-Flavored Vodka (or any fruit flavored vodka)
- Lemon Wedge

Mix, pour over ice, garnish, serve

Daily Exercises for Any Body

Forward Bends - for stretching hamstrings, back, buttocks. Do 4 stretches

The Plank - for all around strength and toning. Work your way up to holding for 60 seconds. Rest for 10 then repeat.

Squats - for quadriceps, hamstrings, inner thighs and buttocks. Do 8 to 12 squats, rest, repeat

Bicycle - for core abdominal strength. Work your way up to a continuous 60 seconds. Rest for 10, then repeat.

Forward Lunges - for quadriceps, hamstrings and buttocks. Do 8 on each side, rest, repeat.

Jumping Jacks - Get your cardio. 1 minute intervals, rest, repeat. Work up to 5 sets of 1 minute intervals.

Don't forget to stretch when you complete the routine.

On those days that you can't get your full work out in, this small routine can get 10 to 15 minutes of exercise in and works all major muscle groups.

Healthy Suggestions From Each Food Group
(remember, it's not rocket science)

Refer to the lists often and add more of your favorite foods to them.

Vegetables - cooked or raw
3 -5, ½ cup servings a day

Kale
Collard Greens
Spinach
Brussel Sprouts
Asparagus
Beets
Tomatoes, cherry
Tomatoes, roma
Summer Squash
Winter Squash
Crook Neck Squash
Zucchini Squash
Peppers, sweet
Carrots
Cauliflower
Artichokes
Eggplant
Okra
Jicama
Snow Peas
Cabbage
Cucumbers
Celery
Lettuce (not Iceburg)
Mushrooms
Radishes
Onions
Sprouts

Fruits
2 - 4, ½ cup servings a day

Raspberries
Blueberries
Blackberries
Strawberries
Watermelon
Cantaloupe
Oranges, all varieties
Tangerine
Apple, all varieties
Apricot
Grapefruit
Cherries
Grapes
Kiwifruit
Mango
Peach
Nectarine
Pear, all varieties
Pineapple
Banana
Papaya
Figs
Honeydew

Protein
2 - 3, 6 oz servings a day

Sardines
Boneless, skinless chicken breast
Boneless, skinless, turkey breast
Lean ground chicken
Lean ground turkey
Fish, fresh water (catfish, tilapia, bass, trout)
Fish, cold water (cod, salmon, tuna)
Game, lean ground (Buffalo, Bison, Venison)
Greek Yogurt, Plain 1%
Shellfish (shrimp, crab, lobster)
Eggs
Clams
Red meat, extra lean
Tofu
Pork Tenderloin
Tuna, canned in water
Turkey, sliced, low-sodium
Ham, sliced, low-sodium
Ricotta Cheese, light
Veggie Burger
Turkey Bacon

Carbohydrates, grains & starches
6 - 11, 1 oz servings a day

Sweet Potatoe
Yams
Quinoa, cooked
Beans (black, red)
Lentils, cooked
Edamame
Peas
Refried Beans, non-fat
Brown rice
Potato, mashed or baked
Corn on the cob
(no, corn is not a vegetable)
Amaranth
Millet
Buckweat
Barley
Bulgur
Oatmeal
Pasta, whole-grain
Couscous, whole-wheat
Crackers, whole-wheat
Bread, whole-grain
Pita Bread, whole-wheat
Waffle, whole-grain
Pancake, whole-grain
English muffin, whole-wheat
Bagel, whole-grain
Tortilla, flour, whole-wheat
Tortilla, corn

Fats
2 - 6, teaspoons a day

Exta-virgin olive oil
Exta-virgin coconut oil
Flaxseed oil
Peanut Butter
Almond Butter
Avacado
Hummus
Pecans
Walnuts
Cashews
Almonds
Peanuts
Olives

Dairy, Cheeses
2 - 3, ½ cup or 4 oz servings a day

Milk, 1%
Milk, skim
Coconut milk
Feta Cheese, crumbled
Goat cheese, crumbled
Mozzarella
Cheddar
Provolone
Monterey Jack
Parmesan
Yogurt
Cottage Cheese, 2%

"No Extra Cost" Foods
unlimited

Water (duh)
Lemon juice Lime juice
Vinegars
Herbs (fresh and dry)
Spices
Galic, cloved, minced
Hot Sauce
Salsa
Flavor Extracts

Follow me on WordPress at: www.reallifeafter40.wordpress.com

Follow me on Pinterest at: www.pinterest.com/pixiesrock247

Follow me on Facebook at: www.facebook.com/RealLifeAfter40

Set Your Goals

_____

_____

_____

_____

_____

_____

_____

_____

Applaud Your Accomplishments

_____

_____

_____

_____

_____